Breastfeeding

A Guide to Breastfeeding your New Born baby

Office on Women's Health

US Department of Health and Human Services

ISBN-13:

978-1499523072

ISBN-10:

1499523076

Breastfeeding

One of the most highly effective preventive measures a mother can take to protect the health of her infant is to breastfeed. However, in the United States, although most mothers hope to breastfeed, and 75% of babies start out being breastfed, only 15% are exclusively breastfed 6 months later. Additionally, rates are significantly lower for African-American infants.

The success rate among mothers who want to breastfeed can be greatly improved through active support from their families, friends, communities, clinicians, health care leaders, employers, and policymakers. Given the importance of breastfeeding for the health and well-being of mothers and children, it is critical that we take action across the country to support breastfeeding.

Why should I breastfeed?

Breastfeeding is normal and healthy for infants and moms. Breast milk has disease-fighting cells called antibodies that help protect infants from germs, illness, and even sudden infant death syndrome (SIDS). Breastfeeding is linked to a lower risk of various health problems for babies, including:

- Ear infections
- Stomach viruses
- Respiratory infections
- Atopic dermatis
- Asthma
- Obesity
- Type 1 and type 2 diabetes
- Childhood leukemia
- Necrotizing enterocolitis, a gastrointestinal disease in preterm infants

Why is breastfeeding important?

In moms, breastfeeding is linked to a lower risk of type 2 diabetes, breast cancer, ovarian cancer, and postpartum depression. Infant formula cannot match the exact chemical makeup of human milk, especially the cells, hormones, and antibodies that fight disease. For most babies, breast milk is easier to digest than formula. It takes time for their stomachs to adjust to digesting proteins in formula because they are made from cow's milk.

How long should I breastfeed?

Many leading health organizations recommend that most infants breastfeed for at least 12 months, with exclusive breastfeeding for the first 6 months. This means that babies are not given any foods or liquids other than breast milk for the first 6 months. These recommendations are supported by organizations including the American Academy of Pediatrics, American Academy of Family Physicians, American College of Obstetricians and Gynecologists, American College of Nurse-Midwives, American Dietetic Association, and American Public Health Association.

Should I supplement with formula?

Giving your baby formula may cause him or her to not want as much breast milk. This will decrease your milk supply. If you are worried that your baby is not eating enough, talk to your baby's doctor.

Does my baby need cereal or water?

Your baby only needs breast milk for the first six months of life. Breast milk alone will provide all the nutrition your baby needs. Giving the baby cereal may cause your baby to not want as much breast milk. This will decrease your milk supply. Even in hot climates, breastfed infants do not need water or juice. When your baby is ready for other foods, they should be iron-rich.

Is it okay for my baby to use a pacifier?

If you want to try it, it is best to wait until the baby is one month old to introduce a pacifier. This allows the baby to learn how to latch well on the breast and get enough to eat.

Is my baby getting enough vitamin D?

Vitamin D is needed to build strong bones. All infants and children should get at least 400 International Units (IU) of vitamin D each day. To meet this need, all breastfed infants (including those supplemented with formula) should be given a vitamin D supplement of 400 IU each day. This should start in the first few days of life. You can buy vitamin D supplements for infants at a drug store or grocery store. Sunlight is a major source of vitamin D, but it is hard to measure how much sunlight your baby gets and too much sun can be harmful. Once your baby is weaned from breast milk, talk to your baby's doctor about whether your baby sill needs vitamin D supplements. Some children do not get enough vitamin D through diet alone.

When should I wean my baby?

The American Academy of Pediatrics recommends breastfeeding beyond the baby's first birthday, and for as long as both the mother and baby would like. The easiest and most natural time to wean is when your child leads the process. But how the mother feels is very important in deciding when to wean.

Is it safe to smoke, drink, or use drugs?

Quit smoking

If you smoke, it is best for you and your baby to quit as soon as possible. If you can't quit, it is still better to breastfeed because it can help protect your baby from respiratory problems and SIDS (sudden infant death syndrome). Be sure to smoke away from your baby and change your clothes to keep your baby away from the chemicals smoking leaves behind. Ask a health care provider for help quitting smoking!

You should avoid alcohol, especially in large amounts. An occasional small drink is ok, but avoid breastfeeding for two hours after the drink.

It is not safe for you to use or be dependent upon an illicit drug. Drugs such as cocaine and marijuana, heroine, and PCP harm your baby. Some reported side effects in babies include seizures, vomiting, poor feeding, and tremors.

Can I take medicines if I am breastfeeding?

Although almost all medicines pass into your milk in small amounts, most have no effect on the baby and can be used while breastfeeding. Very few medicines can't be used while breastfeeding. Discuss any medicines you are using with your doctor and ask before you start using new medicines. This includes prescription and over-the-counter drugs, vitamins, and dietary or herbal supplements. For some women with chronic health problems, stopping a medicine can be more dangerous than the effects it will have on the breastfed baby.

Can I breastfeed if I am sick?

Some women think that when they are sick, they should not breastfeed. But, most common illnesses, such as colds, flu, or diarrhea, can't be passed through breast milk. In fact, if you are sick, your breast milk will have antibodies in it. These antibodies will help protect your baby from getting the same sickness.

Breastfeeding is not advised if the mother:

- Has been infected with HIV or has AIDS. If you have HIV and want to give your baby breast milk, you can contact a human milk bank.

- Is taking antiretroviral medications.

- Has untreated, active tuberculosis.

- Is infected with human T-cell lymphotropic virus type I or type II.

- Is taking prescribed cancer chemotherapy agents, such as antimetabolites, that interfere with DNA replication and cell division.

- Is undergoing radiation therapies; but, such nuclear medicine therapies require only a temporary break from breastfeeding.

What should I do if I have postpartum depression?

Postpartum depression

First, postpartum depression is different than postpartum "blues." The blues — which can include lots of tears, and feeling down and overwhelmed — are common and go away on their own. Postpartum depression is less common, more serious, and can last more than two weeks. Symptoms can include: feeling irritable and sad; having no energy and not being able to sleep; being overly worried about the baby or not having interest in the baby; and feeling worthless and guilty.

If you have postpartum depression, work with your doctor to find the right treatment for you. Treatment may include medication such as antidepressants and talk therapy. Research has shown that while antidepressants pass into breast milk, few problems have been reported in infants. Even so, it is important to let your baby's doctor know if you need to take any medications.

Let your doctor know if your blues do not go away so that you can feel better. If you are having any thoughts about harming yourself or your baby, call 911 right away.

Will my partner be jealous if I breastfeed?

If you prepare your partner in advance, there should be no jealousy. Explain that you need support. Discuss the important and lasting health benefits of breastfeeding. Explain that not making formula means more rest. Be sure to emphasize that breastfeeding can save you money. Your partner can help by changing and burping the baby, sharing chores, and simply sitting with you and the baby to enjoy the special mood that breastfeeding creates. Your partner can also feed the baby pumped breast milk.

Do I have to restrict my sex life while breastfeeding?

No. But, if you are having vaginal dryness, you can try more foreplay and water-based lubricants. You can feed your baby or express some milk before lovemaking so your breasts will be more comfortable and less likely to leak. During sex, you also can put pressure on the nipple when it lets down or have a towel handy to catch the milk.

Do I still need birth control if I am breastfeeding?

Birth control methods

Breastfeeding can delay the return of normal ovulation and menstrual cycles. But, like other forms of birth control, breastfeeding is not a sure way to prevent pregnancy. You should still talk with a health care provider about birth control choices that are okay to use while breastfeeding.

I heard that breast milk can have toxins in it from the environment. Is it still safe for my baby?

While certain chemicals have appeared in breast milk, breastfeeding remains the best way to feed and nurture young infants and children. The advantages of breastfeeding far outweigh any possible risks from environmental pollutants. To date, the effects of such chemicals have only been seen rarely — in babies whose mothers themselves were ill because of them. Infant formula, the water it is mixed with, and/or the bottles or nipples used to give it to the baby can be contaminated with bacteria or chemicals.

Does my breastfed baby need vaccines? Is it safe for me to get a vaccine when I'm breastfeeding?

Yes. Vaccines are very important to your baby's health. Breastfeeding may also enhance your baby's response to certain immunizations, providing more protection. Follow the schedule your doctor gives you and, if you miss any, check with him or her about getting your baby back on track. Breastfeeding while the vaccine is given to your baby — or immediately afterwards — can help relieve pain and sooth an upset baby. Most nursing mothers may also receive vaccines. Breastfeeding does not affect the vaccine. Vaccines are not harmful to your breast milk.

What should I do if my baby bites me?

If your baby starts to clamp down, you can put your finger in the baby's mouth and take him or her off of your breast with a firm, "No." Try not to yell as it may scare the baby. If your baby continues to bite you, you can:

- Stop the feeding right away so the baby is not tempted to get another reaction from you. Don't laugh. This is part of your baby's learning of limits.

- Offer a teething toy, or a snack (if older baby), or a drink from a cup instead.

- Put your baby down for a moment to show that biting brings a negative consequence. You can then pick your baby up again to give comfort.

What do I do if my baby keeps crying?

If your baby does not seem comforted by breastfeeding or other soothing measures, talk to your baby's doctor. Your baby may have colic or may be uncomfortable or in pain. You can also check to see if your baby is teething. The doctor and a lactation consultant can help you find ways to help your baby eat well.

Breastfeeding

Why breastfeeding is important

- Breastfeeding protects babies
- Mothers benefit from breastfeeding
- Breastfeeding benefits society
- Breastfeeding during an emergency
- More information on why breastfeeding is important

Breastfeeding protects babies

1. **Early breast milk is liquid gold** – Known as liquid gold, colostrum (coh-LOSS-trum) is the thick yellow first breast milk that you make during pregnancy and just after birth. This milk is very rich in nutrients and antibodies to protect your baby. Although your baby only gets a small amount of colostrum at each feeding, it matches the amount his or her tiny stomach can hold.

2. **Your breast milk changes as your baby grows** – Colostrum changes into what is called mature milk. By the third to fifth day after birth, this mature breast milk has just the right amount of fat, sugar, water, and protein to help your baby continue to grow. It is a thinner type of milk than colostrum, but it provides all of the nutrients and antibodies your baby needs.

3. **Breast milk is easier to digest** – For most babies — especially premature babies — breast milk is easier to

12

digest than formula. The proteins in formula are made from cow's milk and it takes time for babies' stomachs to adjust to digesting them.

4. **Breast milk fights disease** – The cells, hormones, and antibodies in breast milk protect babies from illness. This protection is unique; formula cannot match the chemical makeup of human breast milk. In fact, among formula-fed babies, ear infections and diarrhea are more common. Formula-fed babies also have higher risks of:

   o Necrotizing (nek-roh-TEYE-zing) enterocolitis (en-TUR-oh-coh-lyt-iss), a disease that affects the gastrointestinal tract in preterm infants.

   o Lower respiratory infections

   o Asthma

   o Obesity

   o Type 2 diabetes

Some research shows that breastfeeding can also reduce the risk of Type 1 diabetes, childhood leukemia, and atopic dermatitis (a type of skin rash) in babies. Breastfeeding has also been shown to lower the risk of SIDS (sudden infant death syndrome).

Did you know?

While formula-feeding raises health risks in babies, it can also save lives. Very rarely, babies are born unable to tolerate milk of any kind. These babies must have soy formula. Formula may also be needed if the mother has certain health conditions and she does not have access to donor breast milk. To learn more about rare breastfeeding restrictions in the mother, visit the Breastfeeding a baby with health problems section..

Mothers benefit from breastfeeding

1. **Life can be easier when you breastfeed** – Breastfeeding may take a little more effort than formula feeding at first. But it can make life easier once you and your baby settle into a good routine. Plus, when you breastfeed, there are no bottles and nipples to sterilize. You do not have to buy, measure, and mix formula. And there are no bottles to warm in the middle of the night! You can satisfy your baby's hunger right away when breastfeeding.

2. **Breastfeeding can save money** – Formula and feeding supplies can cost well over $1,500 each year, depending on how much your baby eats. Breastfed babies are also sick less often, which can lower health care costs.

3. **Breastfeeding can feel great** – Physical contact is important to newborns. It can help them feel more secure, warm, and comforted. Mothers can benefit from this closeness, as well. Breastfeeding requires a mother to take some quiet relaxed time to bond. The skin-to-skin contact can boost the mother's oxytocin (OKS-ee-TOH-suhn) levels. Oxytocin is a hormone that helps milk flow and can calm the mother.

4. **Breastfeeding can be good for the mother's health, too** – Breastfeeding is linked to a lower risk of these health problems in women:

    1. Type 2 diabetes

    2. Breast cancer

    3. Ovarian cancer

4. Postpartum depression

Experts are still looking at the effects of breastfeeding on osteoporosis and weight loss after birth. Many studies have reported greater weight loss for breastfeeding mothers than for those who don't. But more research is needed to understand if a strong link exists.

5. **Mothers miss less work** – Breastfeeding mothers miss fewer days from work because their infants are sick less often.

Breastfeeding benefits society

The nation benefits overall when mothers breastfeed. Recent research shows that if 90 percent of families breastfed exclusively for 6 months, nearly 1,000 deaths among infants could be prevented. The United States would also save $13 billion per year — medical care costs are lower for fully breastfed infants than never-breastfed infants. Breastfed infants typically need fewer sick care visits, prescriptions, and hospitalizations.

Breastfeeding also contributes to a more productive workforce since mothers miss less work to care for sick infants. Employer medical costs are also lower.

Breastfeeding is also better for the environment. There is less trash and plastic waste compared to that produced by formula cans and bottle supplies.

Breastfeeding during an emergency

When an emergency occurs, breastfeeding can save lives:

- Breastfeeding protects babies from the risks of a contaminated water supply.

- Breastfeeding can help protect against respiratory illnesses and diarrhea. These diseases can be fatal in populations displaced by disaster.

- Breast milk is the right temperature for babies and helps to prevent hypothermia, when the body temperature drops too low.

- Breast milk is readily available without needing other supplies.

Learning to breastfeed

- How breast milk is made
- What you can do before you give birth
- Tips for getting off to a good start
- Bringing your baby to the breast to latch
- How often should I breastfeed? How long should feedings be?
- Breastfeeding holds
- Tips for making it work
- Making plenty of milk
- How to know your baby is getting enough milk
- How long should I breastfeed?

Keep in mind that breastfeeding is a learned skill. It requires patience and practice. For some women, the learning stages can be frustrating and uncomfortable. And some situations make breastfeeding even harder, such as babies born early or health problems in the mother. The good news is that it will get easier, and support for breastfeeding mothers is growing. Keep in mind that you make milk in response to your baby sucking at the breast. The more milk your baby removes from the breasts, the more milk you will make.

How breast milk is made

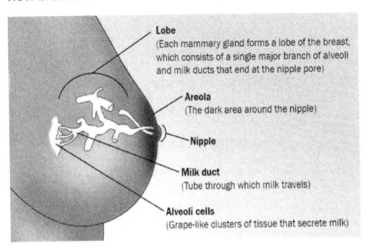

Lobe
(Each mammary gland forms a lobe of the breast, which consists of a single major branch of alveoli and milk ducts that end at the nipple pore)

Areola
(The dark area around the nipple)

Nipple

Milk duct
(Tube through which milk travels)

Alveoli cells
(Grape-like clusters of tissue that secrete milk)

Knowing how the breast works to produce milk can help you understand the breastfeeding process. The breast itself is a gland that is made up of several parts, including:

- **Glandular tissue** – body tissue that makes and releases one or more substances for use in the body. Some glands make fluids that affect tissues or organs. Others make hormones or assist with blood production. In the breast, this tissue is involved in milk production.

- **Connective tissue** – a type of body tissue that supports other tissues and binds them together. This tissue provides support in the breast.

- **Blood** – fluid in the body made up of plasma, red and white blood cells, and platelets. Blood carries oxygen and nutrients to and waste materials away from all body tissues. In the breast, blood nourishes the breast tissue and provides nutrients needed for milk production.

- **Lymph** – the almost colorless fluid that travels through the lymphatic system and carries cells that help fight infection and disease. Lymph tissue in the breast helps remove waste.

- **Nerves** – cells that are the building blocks of the nervous system (the system that records and transmits information chemically and electrically within a person). Nerve tissue in the breast makes breasts sensitive to touch, allowing the baby's sucking to stimulate the let-down or milk-ejection reflex and milk production.

- **Fatty tissue** – connective tissue that contains stored fat. It is also known as adipose tissue. Fatty tissue in the breast protects the breast from injury. Fatty tissue is what mostly affects the size of a woman's breast. Breast size does not have an effect on the amount of milk or the quality of milk a woman makes.

Special cells inside your breasts make milk. These cells are called alveoli (al-VEE-uh-leye). When your breasts become fuller and tender during pregnancy, this is a sign that the alveoli are getting ready to work. Some women do not feel these changes in their breasts. Others may sense these changes after their baby is born.

The alveoli make milk in response to the hormone prolactin (proh-LAK-tin). Prolactin rises when the baby suckles. Another hormone, oxytocin (oks-ee-TOH-suhn), causes small muscles around the cells to contract and move the milk through a series of small tubes called milk ducts. This moving of the milk is called let-down reflex.

Oxytocin also causes the muscles of the uterus to contract during and after birth. This helps the uterus to get back to its original size. It also lessens any bleeding a woman may have after giving birth. The release of both prolactin and oxytocin may be responsible in part for a mother's intense feeling of needing to be with her baby.

What is a let-down reflex?

A let-down reflex or milk ejection reflex is a conditioned reflex ejecting milk from the alveoli through the ducts to the sinuses of the breast and the nipple. This reflex makes it easier to breastfeed your baby. Let-down happens a few seconds to several minutes after you start breastfeeding your baby. It can happen a few times during a feeding, too. You may feel a tingle in your breast or you may feel a little uncomfortable. Keep in mind that some women don't feel anything. Let-down can happen at other times, too, such as when you hear your baby cry or when you may just be thinking about your baby. If your milk lets down as more of a gush and it bothers your baby, try expressing some milk by hand before you start breastfeeding.

What you can do before you give birth

What dad can do

A woman who is thinking about how to feed her baby values her partner's advice. A father's approval and support of breastfeeding can boost the mother's confidence and help her to overcome challenges. But supporting a woman's choice to breastfeed is not the father's only role. Although the bond between mother and baby is important, so is the bond between father and baby. Babies need cuddles and hugs from their dads, too! In fact, skin-to-skin contact helps baby and father bond much like it does for mother and baby.

To prepare for breastfeeding, the most important thing you can do is have confidence in yourself. Committing to breastfeeding starts with the belief that you can do it!

Other steps you can take to prepare for breastfeeding:

1. Get good prenatal care, which can help you avoid early delivery. Babies born too early often need special care, which can make breastfeeding harder.

2. Tell your health care provider about your plans to breastfeed, and ask if the place where you plan to deliver your baby has the staff and set-up to support successful breastfeeding. Some hospitals and birth centers have taken special steps to create the best possible environment for successful breastfeeding. They are called Baby-Friendly Hospitals and Birth Centers. Women who deliver in a baby-friendly facility are promised the information and support they need to breastfeed their infants.

3. Take a breastfeeding class. Pregnant women who learn about how to breastfeed are more likely to be successful than those who do not. Breastfeeding classes offer pregnant women and their partners the chance to prepare and ask questions before the baby's arrival.

4. Ask your health care provider to recommend a lactation consultant. You can establish a relationship before the baby comes, or be ready if you need help after the baby is born.

5. Talk to your health care provider about your health. Discuss any breast surgery or injury you may have had. If you have depression or are taking medications, discuss treatment options that can work with breastfeeding.

6. Tell your health care provider that you would like to breastfeed your newborn baby as soon as possible after delivery. The sucking instinct is very strong within the first hour of life.

7. Talk to friends who have breastfed or consider joining a breastfeeding support group.

8. Talk to fathers, partners, and other family members about how they can help. Partners and family members can:

   o Support the breastfeeding relationship by being kind and encouraging.

   o Show their love and appreciation for all of the work that is put into breastfeeding.

   o Be good listeners when a mother needs to talk through breastfeeding concerns.

   o Make sure the mother has enough to drink and gets enough rest, help around the house, and take care of other children at home.

   o Give emotional nourishment to the child through playing and cuddling.

Tips for getting off to a good start

After you have the baby, these steps can help you get off to a great start:

- Breastfeed as soon as possible after birth.

- Ask for an on-site lactation consultant to come help you.

- Ask the staff not to give your baby other food or formula, unless it is medically necessary.

- Allow your baby to stay in your hospital room all day and night so that you can breastfeed often. Or, ask the nurses to bring you your baby for feedings.

- Try to avoid giving your baby any pacifiers or artificial nipples so that he or she gets used to latching onto just your breast.

Bringing your baby to the breast to latch

Did you know?

Some babies latch on right away and, for some, it takes more time.

When awake, your baby will move his or her head back and forth, looking and feeling for the breast with his or her mouth and lips. The steps below can help you get your baby to "latch" on to the breast to start eating. Keep in mind that there is no one way to start breastfeeding. As long as the baby is latched on well, how you get there is up to you.

- Hold your baby, wearing only a diaper, against your bare chest. Hold the baby upright with his or her head under your chin. Your baby will be comfortable in that cozy valley between your breasts. You can ask your partner or a nurse to place a blanket across your baby's back and bring your bedcovers over you both. Your skin temperature will rise to warm your baby.

- Support his or her neck and shoulders with one hand and hips with the other. He or she may move in an effort to find your breast.

- Your baby's head should be tilted back slightly to make it easy to suck and swallow. With his or her head back and mouth open, the tongue is naturally down and ready for the breast to go on top of it.

- Allow your breast to hang naturally. When your baby feels it with his or her cheek, he or she may open his or her mouth wide and reach it up and over the nipple. You can also guide the baby to latch on as you see in the illustrations below.

- At first, your baby's nose will be lined up opposite your nipple. As his or her chin presses into your breast, his or her wide, open mouth will get a large mouthful of breast for a deep latch. Keep in mind that your baby can breathe at the breast. The nostrils flare to allow air in.

- Do not put your hands on your baby's head. As it tilts back, support your baby's upper back and shoulders with the palm of your hand and pull your baby in close.

Getting your baby to latch

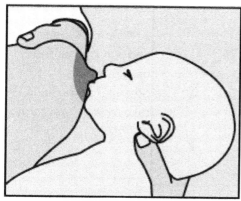

1. Tickle the baby's lips to encourage him or her to open wide.

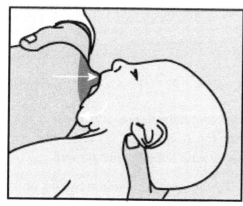

2. Pull your baby close so that the chin and lower jaw moves into your breast first.

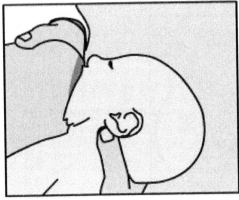

3. Watch the lower lip and aim it as far from base of nipple as possible, so the baby takes a large mouthful of breast.

Signs of a good latch

Did you know?

A good latch is important for your baby to breastfeed effectively and for your comfort. During the early days of breastfeeding, it can take time and patience for your baby to latch on well.

- The latch feels comfortable to you, without hurting or pinching. How it feels is more important than how it looks.

- Your baby's chest is against your body and he or she does not have to turn his or her head while drinking.

- You see little or no areola, depending on the size of your areola and the size of your baby's mouth. If areola is showing, you will see more above your baby's lip and less below.

- When your baby is positioned well, his or her mouth will be filled with breast.

- The tongue is cupped under the breast, although you might not see it.

- You hear or see your baby swallow. Some babies swallow so quietly, a pause in their breathing may be the only sign of swallowing.

- You see the baby's ears "wiggle" slightly.

- Your baby's lips turn out like fish lips, not in. You may not even be able to see the bottom lip.

- Your baby's chin touches your breast.

Help with latch problems

Are you in pain? Many moms report that their breasts can be tender at first until both they and their baby find comfortable breastfeeding positions and a good latch. Once you have done this, breastfeeding should be comfortable. If it hurts, your baby may be sucking on only the nipple. Gently break your baby's suction to your breast by placing a clean finger in the corner of your baby's mouth and try again. Also, your nipple should not look flat or compressed when it comes out of your baby's mouth. It should look round and long, or the same shape as it was before the feeding.

Are you or your baby frustrated? Take a short break and hold your baby in an upright position. Try holding him or her between your breasts skin-to-skin. Talk, sing, or provide your finger for sucking for comfort. Try to breastfeed again in a little while. Or, the baby may start moving to the breast on his or her own from this position.

Does your baby have a weak suck, or make only tiny suckling movements? Break your baby's suction and try again. He or she may not have a deep enough latch to remove the milk from your breast. Talk with a lactation consultant or pediatrician if your baby's suck feels weak or if you are not sure he or she is getting enough milk. Rarely, a health problem causes the weak suck.

How often should I breastfeed? How long should feedings be?

Early and often! Breastfeed as soon as possible after birth, then breastfeed at least 8 to 12 times every 24 hours to make plenty of milk for your baby. This means that in the first few days after birth, your baby will likely need to breastfeed about every hour or two in the daytime and a couple of times at night. Healthy babies develop their own feeding schedules. Follow your baby's cues for when he or she is ready to eat.

Feedings may be 15 to 20 minutes or longer per breast. But there is no set time. Your baby will let you know when he or she is finished. If you are worried that your baby is not eating enough, talk to your baby's doctor.

Breastfeeding holds

Some moms find that the following positions are helpful ways to get comfortable and support their babies in finding a good latch. You also can use pillows under your arms, elbows, neck, or back to give you added comfort and support. Keep in mind that what works well for one feeding may not work well for the next. Keep trying different positions until you are comfortable.

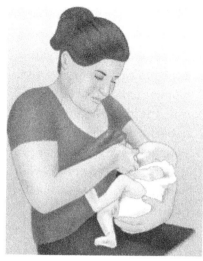

Cradle hold – An easy, common hold that is comfortable for most mothers and babies. Hold your baby with his or her head on your forearm and his or her whole body facing yours.

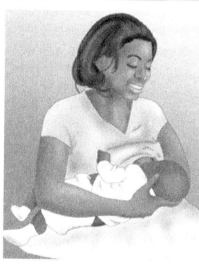

Cross cradle or transitional hold – Useful for premature babies or babies with a weak suck because it gives extra head support and may help babies stay latched. Hold your baby along the opposite arm from the breast you are using. Support your baby's head with the palm of your hand at the base of his or her neck.

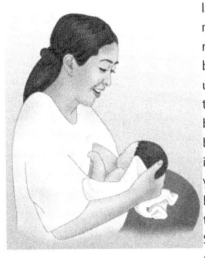

Clutch or "football" hold – Useful for mothers who had a c-section and mothers with large breasts, flat or inverted nipples, or a strong letdown reflex. It is also helpful for babies who prefer to be more upright. This hold allows you to better see and control your baby's head, and keep the baby away from a c-section incision. Hold your baby at your side, lying on his or her back, with his or her head at the level of your nipple. Support baby's head with the palm of your hand at the base of the head. (The baby is placed almost under the arm.)

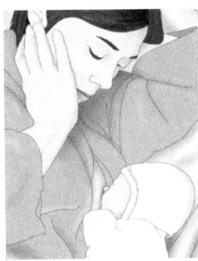

Side-lying position – Useful for mothers who had a c-section or to help any mother get extra rest while the baby breastfeeds. Lie on your side with your baby facing you. Pull your baby close so your baby faces your body.

Tips for making it work

1. **Learn your baby's hunger signs** – When babies are hungry, they become more alert and active. They may put their hands or fists to their mouths, make sucking motions with their mouth, or turn their heads looking for the breast. If anything touches the baby's cheek — such as a hand — the baby may turn towards this hand, ready to eat. This sign of hunger is called rooting. Offer your breast when your baby shows rooting signs. Crying can be a late sign of hunger and it may be harder to latch once the baby is upset. Over time, you will be able to learn your baby's cues for when to start feeding.

2. **Follow your baby's lead** – Make sure you are both comfortable and follow your baby's lead after he or she is latched on well. Some babies take both breasts at each feeding. Other babies only take one breast at a feeding. Help your baby finish the first breast, as long as he or she is still sucking and swallowing. This will ensure the baby gets the "hind" milk — the fattier milk at the end of a feeding. Your baby will let go of the breast when he or she is finished, and often falls asleep. Offer the other breast if he or she seems to want more.

3. **Keep your baby close to you** – Remember that your baby is not used to this new world and needs to be held very close to his or her mother. Being skin-to-skin helps babies cry less and stabilizes the baby's heart and breathing rates.

4. **Avoid nipple confusion** – Avoid using pacifiers, bottles, and supplements of infant formula in the first few weeks unless there is a medical reason to do so. If supplementation is needed, try to give expressed breast milk first. But it's best just to feed at the breast. This will

help you make milk and keep your baby from getting confused while learning to breastfeed.

5. **Sleep safely and close by** – Have your baby sleep in a crib or bassinet in your room, so that you can breastfeed more easily at night. Sharing a room with parents is linked to a lower risk of SIDS (sudden infant death syndrome).

6. **Know when to wake the baby** – In the early weeks after birth, you should wake your baby to feed if 4 hours have passed since the beginning of the last feeding. Some tips for waking the baby include:

   o Changing your baby's diaper

   o Placing your baby skin-to-skin

   o Massaging your baby's back, abdomen, and legs

If your baby is falling asleep at the breast during most feedings, talk to the baby's doctor about a weight check. Also, see a lactation consultant to make sure the baby is latching on well.

Making plenty of milk

Your breasts will easily make and supply milk directly in response to your baby's needs. The more often and effectively a baby breastfeeds, the more milk will be made. Babies are trying to double their weight in a few short months, and their tummies are small, so they need many feedings to grow and to be healthy.

Most mothers can make plenty of milk for their baby. If you think you have a low milk supply, talk to a lactation consultant.

What will happen with you, your baby, and your milk in the

first few weeks

Time	Milk	The baby	You (Mom)
Birth	Your body makes colostrum (a rich, thick, yellowish milk) in small amounts. It gives your baby a healthy dose of early protection against diseases.	Will probably be awake in the first hour after birth. This is a good time to breastfeed your baby.	You will be tired and excited.
First 12-24 hours	Your baby will drink about 1 teaspoon of colostrum at each feeding. You may or may not see the colostrum, but it has what the	It is normal for the baby to sleep heavily. Labor and delivery are hard work! Some babies like to nuzzle and may be too sleepy to latch well at first. Feedings may be short and	You will be tired, too. Be sure to rest.

	baby needs and in the right amount.	disorganized. As your baby wakes up, take advantage of your baby's strong instinct to suck and feed every 1-2 hours. Many babies like to eat or lick, pause, savor, doze, then eat again.	
Next 3-5 days	Your white milk comes in. It is normal for it to have a yellow or golden tint first. Talk to a doctor and lactation consultant if your milk is not yet in.	Your baby will feed a lot (this helps your breasts make plenty of milk), at least 8-12 times or more in 24 hours. Very young breastfed babies don't eat on a schedule. Because breast milk is more easily digested than formula, breastfed babies eat more often than formula-fed babies. It is okay	Your breasts may feel full and leak. (You can use disposable or cloth pads in your bra to help with leaking.)

if your baby eats every 2-3 hours for several hours, then sleeps for 3-4 hours. Feedings may take about 15-20 minutes on each side. The baby's sucking rhythm will be slow and long. You might hear gulping.

| The first 4-6 weeks | White breast milk continues. | Your baby will likely be better at breastfeeding and have a larger stomach to hold more milk. Feedings may take less time and will be farther apart. | Your body gets used to breastfeeding so your breasts will be softer and the leaking may slow down. |

How to know your baby is getting enough milk

Many babies, but not all, lose a small amount of weight in the first days after birth. Your baby's doctor will check his or her weight at your first visit after you leave the hospital. Make sure to visit your baby's doctor within three to five days after birth and then again at two to three weeks of age for check-ups.

You can tell if your baby is getting plenty of milk if he or she is mostly content and gaining weight steadily after the first week of age. From birth to three months, typical weight gain is two-thirds to one ounce each day.

Other signs that your baby is getting plenty of milk:

- He or she is passing enough clear or pale yellow urine, and it's not deep yellow or orange (see the chart below).

- He or she has enough bowel movements (see the chart below).

- He or she switches between short sleeping periods and wakeful, alert periods.

- He or she is satisfied and content after feedings.

- Your breasts feel softer after you feed your baby.

Talk to your baby's doctor if you are worried that your baby is not eating enough.

How much do babies typically eat?

A newborn's tummy is very small, especially in the early days. Once breastfeeding is established, exclusively breastfed babies from 1 to 6 months of age take in between 19 and 30 ounces per day. If you breastfeed 8 times per day, the baby would eat around 3 ounces per feeding. Older babies will take less breastmilk as other food is introduced. Every baby is different, though.

The newborn tummy

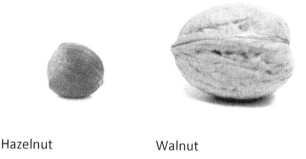

Hazelnut   Walnut

At birth, the baby's stomach can comfortably digest what would fit in a hazelnut (about 1-2 teaspoons). In the first week, the baby's stomach grows to hold about 2 ounces or what would fit in a walnut.

Minimum number of wet diapers and bowel movements in a baby's first week
(it is fine if your baby has more) 1 day = 24 hours

Baby's age	Number of wet diapers	Number of bowel movements	Color and texture of bowel movements

Day			
Day 1 (first 24 hours after birth)	1	The first one usually occurs within 8 hours after birth	Thick, tarry, and black
Day 2	2	3	Thick, tarry, and black
Day 3	5-6	3	Looser greenish to yellow (color may vary)
Day 4	6	3	Yellow, soft, and watery
Day 5	6	3	Loose and seedy, yellow color
Day 6	6	3	Loose and seedy, yellow color
Day 7	6	3	Larger amounts of loose and seedy, yellow color

How long should I breastfeed?

Many leading health organizations recommend that most infants breastfeed for at least 12 months, with exclusive breastfeeding for the first six months. This means that babies are not given any foods or liquids other than breast milk for the first six months. These recommendations are supported by organizations including the American Academy of Pediatrics, American Academy of Family Physicians, American Congress of Obstetricians and Gynecologists, American College of Nurse-

Midwives, American Dietetic Association, and American Public Health Association.

CPSIA information can be obtained at www.ICGtesting.com
Printed in the USA
LVOW04s0307070915

453092LV00031B/983/P

9 781499 523072